My Helping Hands

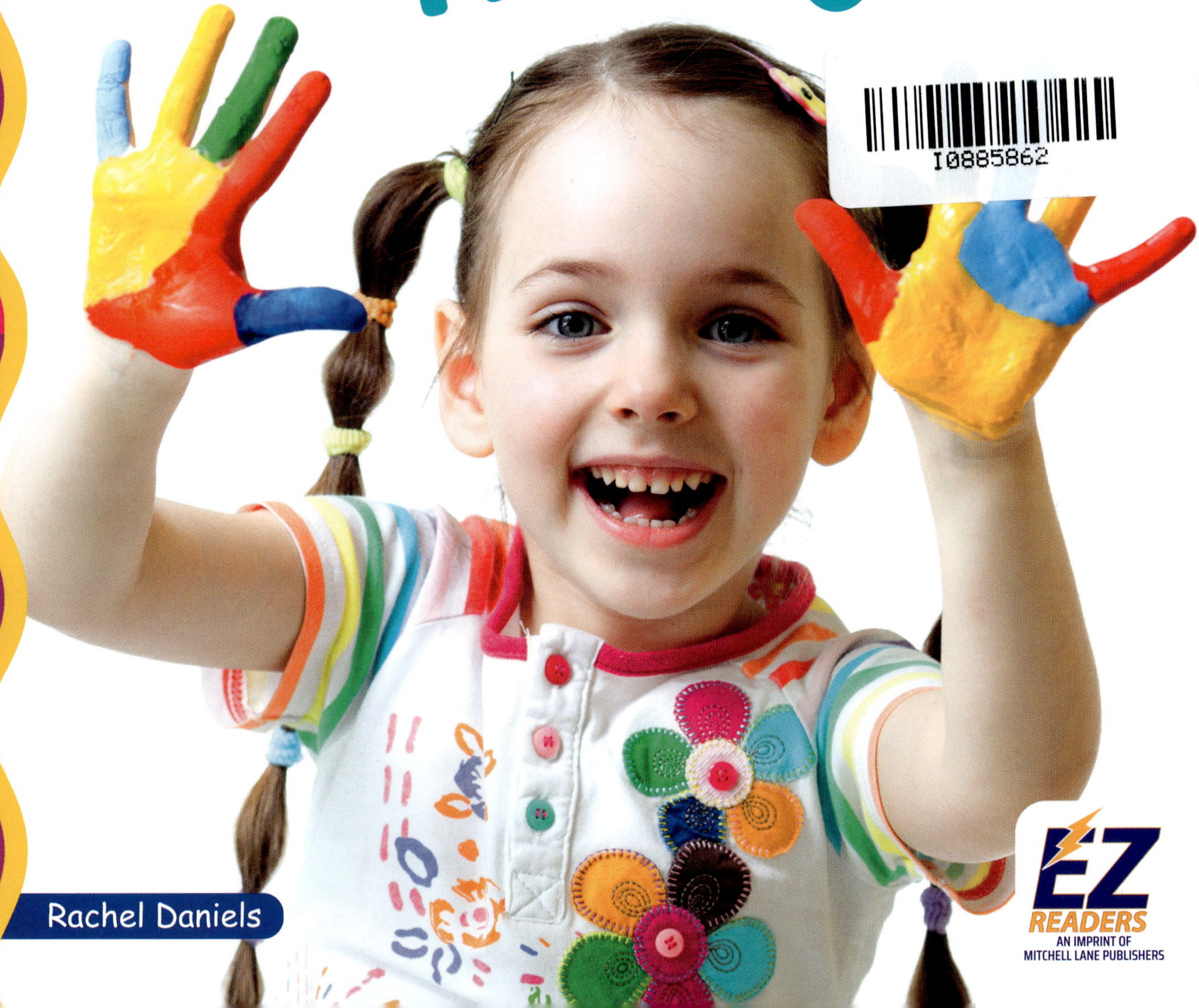

Rachel Daniels

EZ READERS
AN IMPRINT OF
MITCHELL LANE PUBLISHERS

CREATING YOUNG NONFICTION READERS

EZ Readers offer nonfiction for beginning readers in PreK through first grade, using simple language, clear illustrations, and engaging facts to build vocabulary and confidence.

TIPS FOR READING NONFICTION WITH BEGINNING READERS

Talk about Nonfiction

Begin by explaining that nonfiction books give us information that is true. The book will be organized around a specific topic or idea, and we may learn new facts through reading.

Look at the Parts

Most nonfiction books have helpful features. Our *EZ Readers* include color photographs and graphic aids, a table of contents, a glossary, and an index. Share the purpose of these features with your reader.

Color Photos and Graphic Aids

A lot of information can be found by "reading" photos, charts, maps, and other graphic aids found within nonfiction texts. Help your reader learn more about the different ways information can be displayed.

Table of Contents

Located at the front of the book, this list shows the big ideas within the text and the page numbers where they can be found.

Glossary

Located at the back of the book, the glossary defines key words and phrases that are related to the topic. These words and phrases can be found in the text in colored type.

Index

Located at the back of the book, an index is an alphabetical list of topics and the page numbers where they can be found.

With a little help and guidance about reading nonfiction, you can feel good about introducing a young reader to the world of *EZ Readers* nonfiction books.

EZ Readers is an imprint of:

Mitchell Lane
PUBLISHERS

2001 SW 31st Avenue
Hallandale, FL 33009
mitchelllanepub.com

First Edition, 2026.

Author: Rachel Daniels
Editor: Morgan Brody

ISBN 979-8-89260-828-2 (library binding)
ISBN 979-8-90145-034-5 (paperback)
ISBN 979-8-89260-831-2 (ebook)

LC record available at https://lccn.loc.gov/2025950842

Photo credits: Shutterstock, Alex Konon, cover, 1, 2, 3, 7, 16, 20; yusuf_demirci, cover, 1; Oksana Kuzmina, cover, 1; Roman Samborskyi, 5; Sajjad Farooq, 5, 22; Maryshot, 6; PH888, 8–9, 22; Rawpixels stock, 10, 22; Kdonmuang, 10, 22; Poznyakov, 12–13; pics five, 14, 22; Pressmaster, 17, 22; Shutterstock, 18–19; Hung Chung Chih, 21; Freepik, Designed by starline, 3, 5, 8,13,15

Table of Contents

Busy Hands

My hands wave hello.

They clap, clap, clap.

My hands stay busy all day!

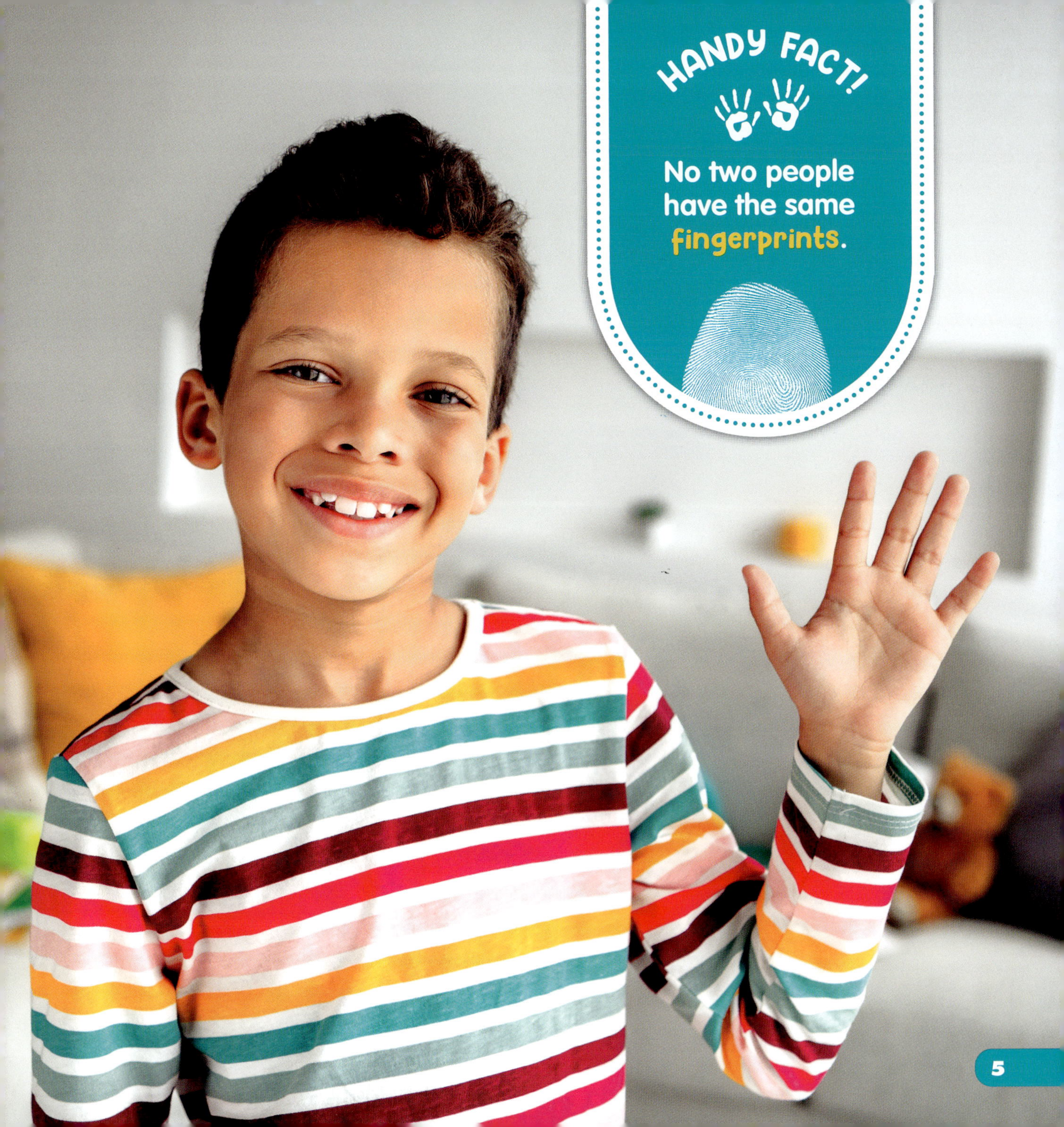

HANDY FACT!

No two people have the same **fingerprints**.

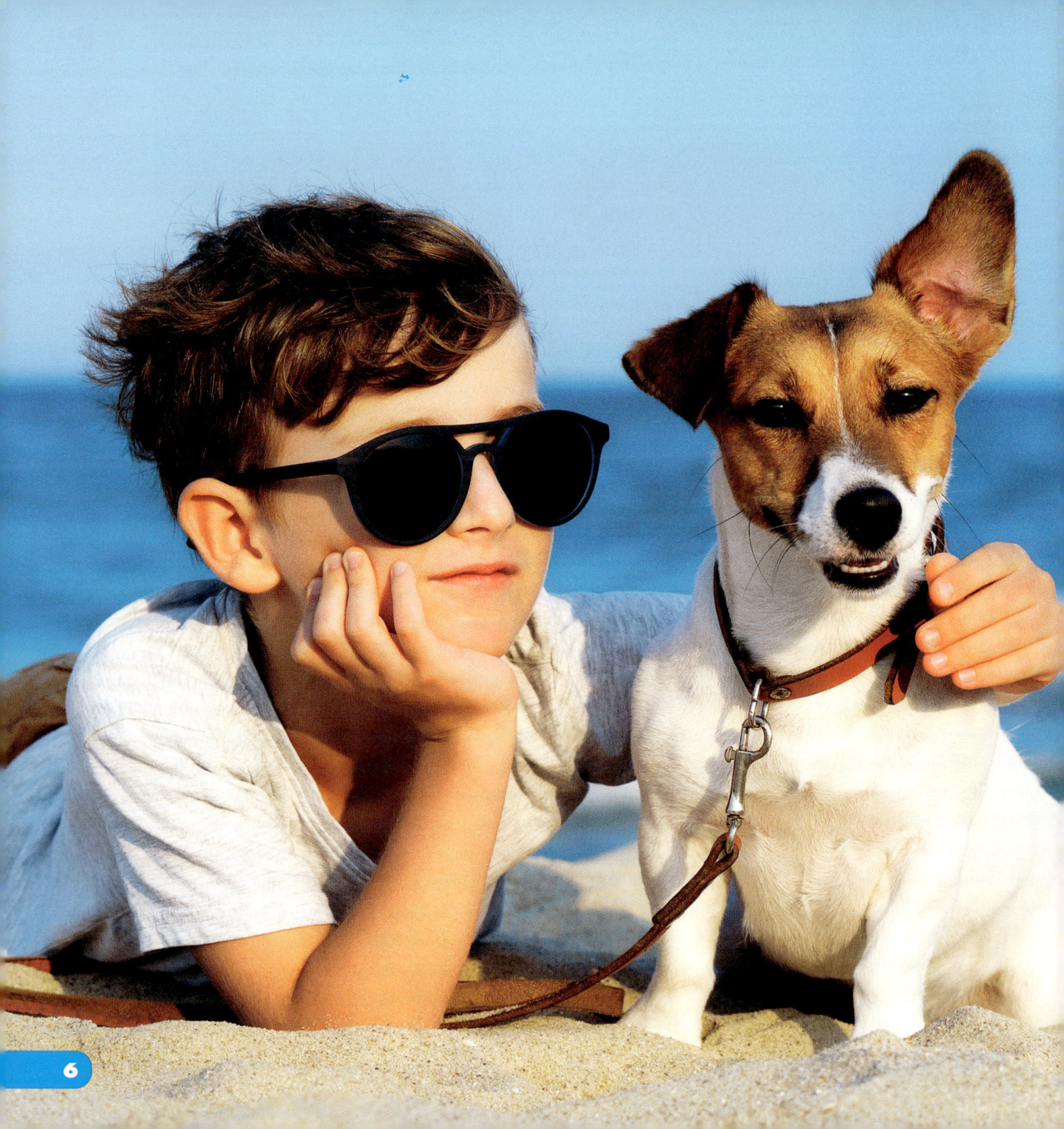

Touch and Feel

Hands feel soft fur.

They touch hot and cold.

My hands hold books.

They **carry** toys.

My helping hands
keep things safe.

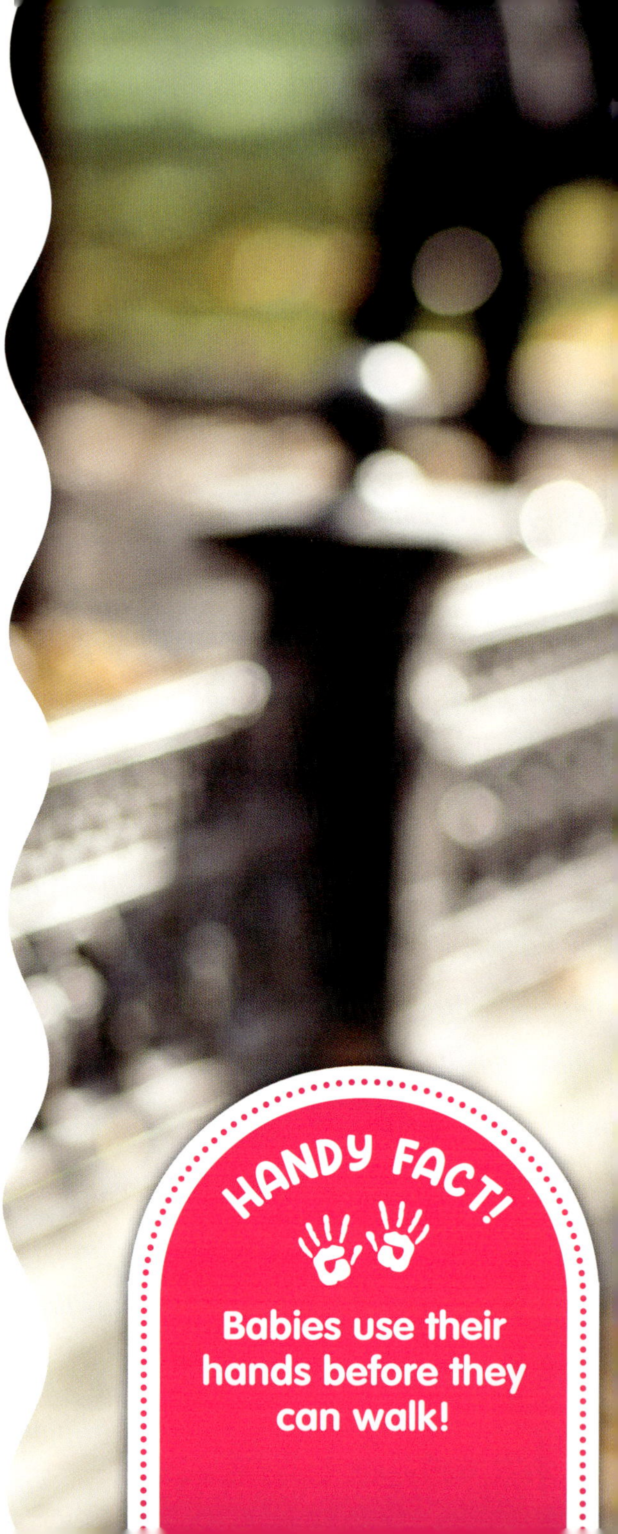

HANDY FACT!

Babies use their hands before they can walk!

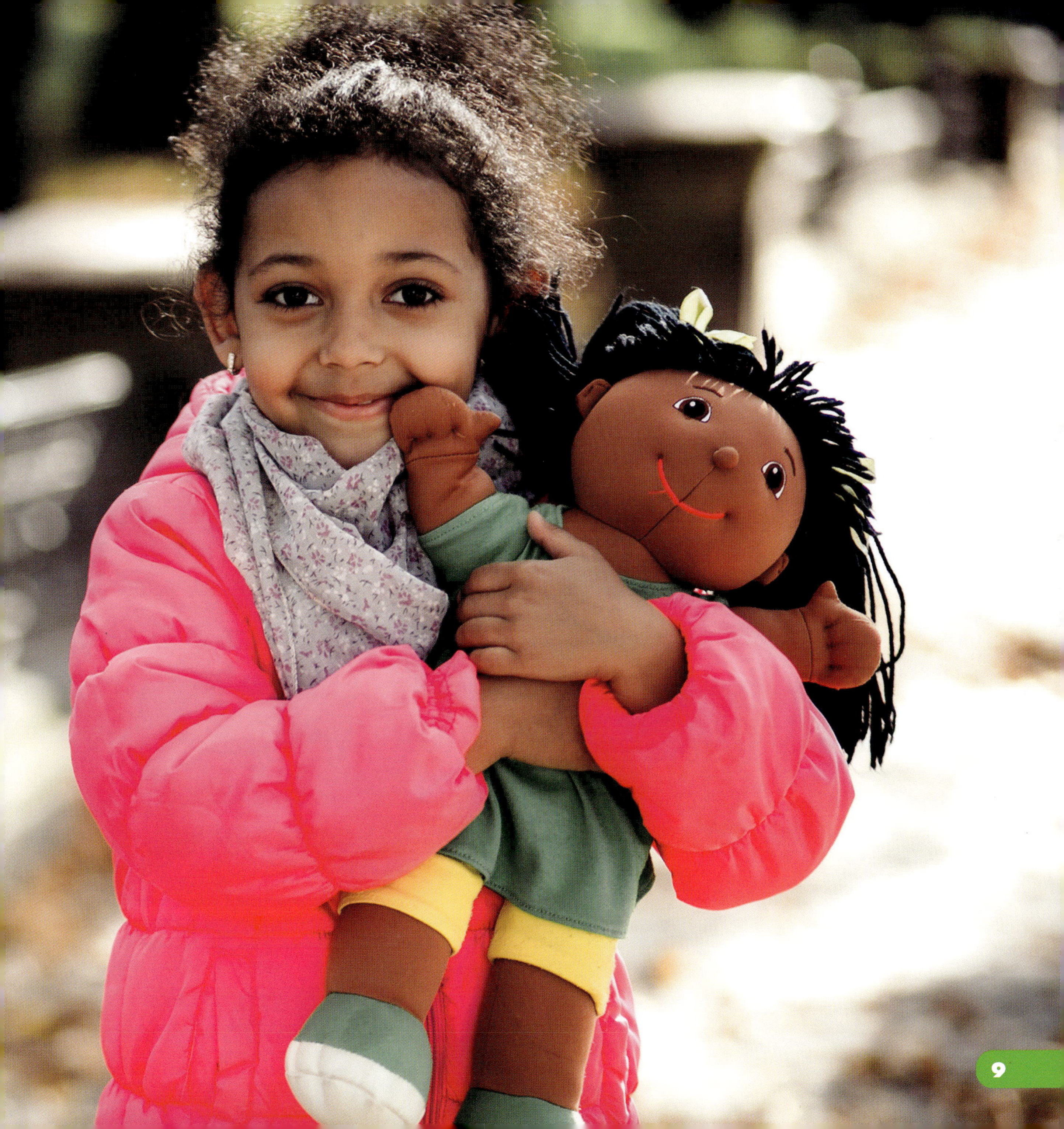

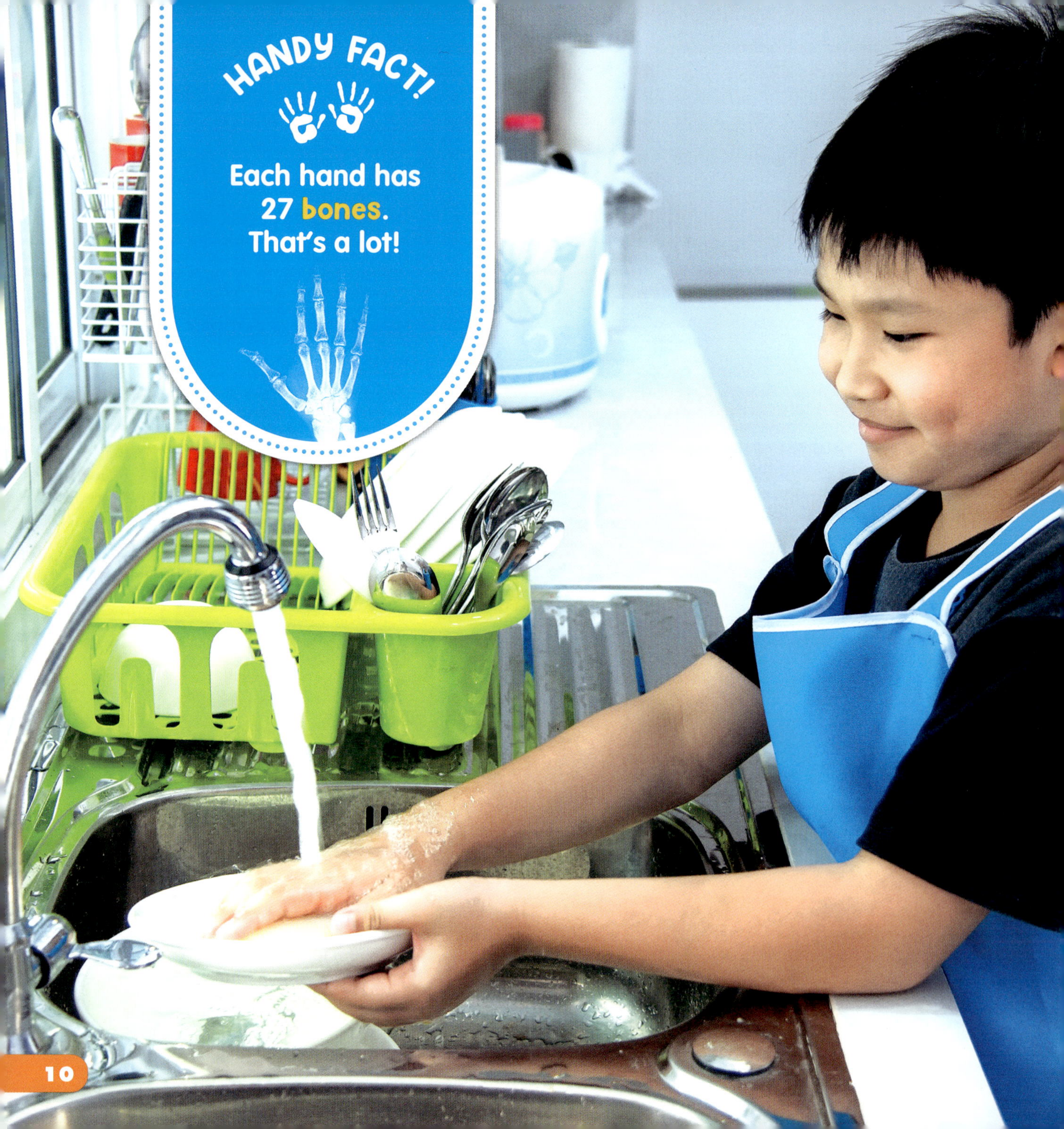

HANDY FACT!

Each hand has 27 **bones**. That's a lot!

Hands wash dishes.

Hands pick up blocks.

My helping hands
clean and **share**.

My hands draw and paint.

They build and play.

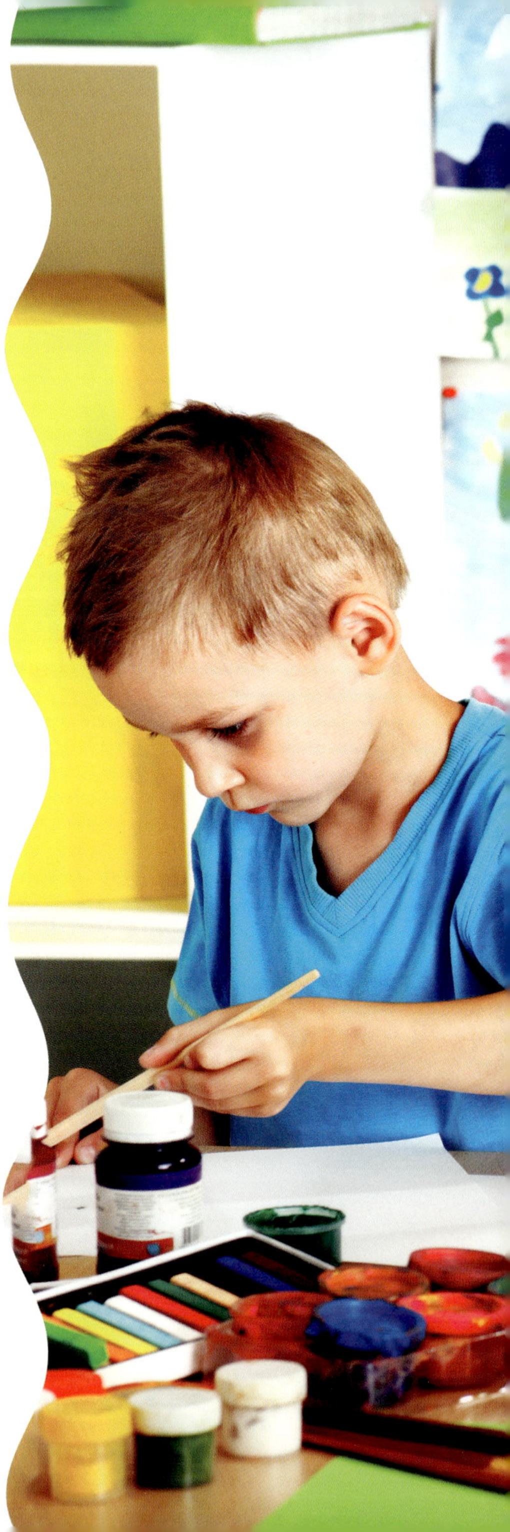

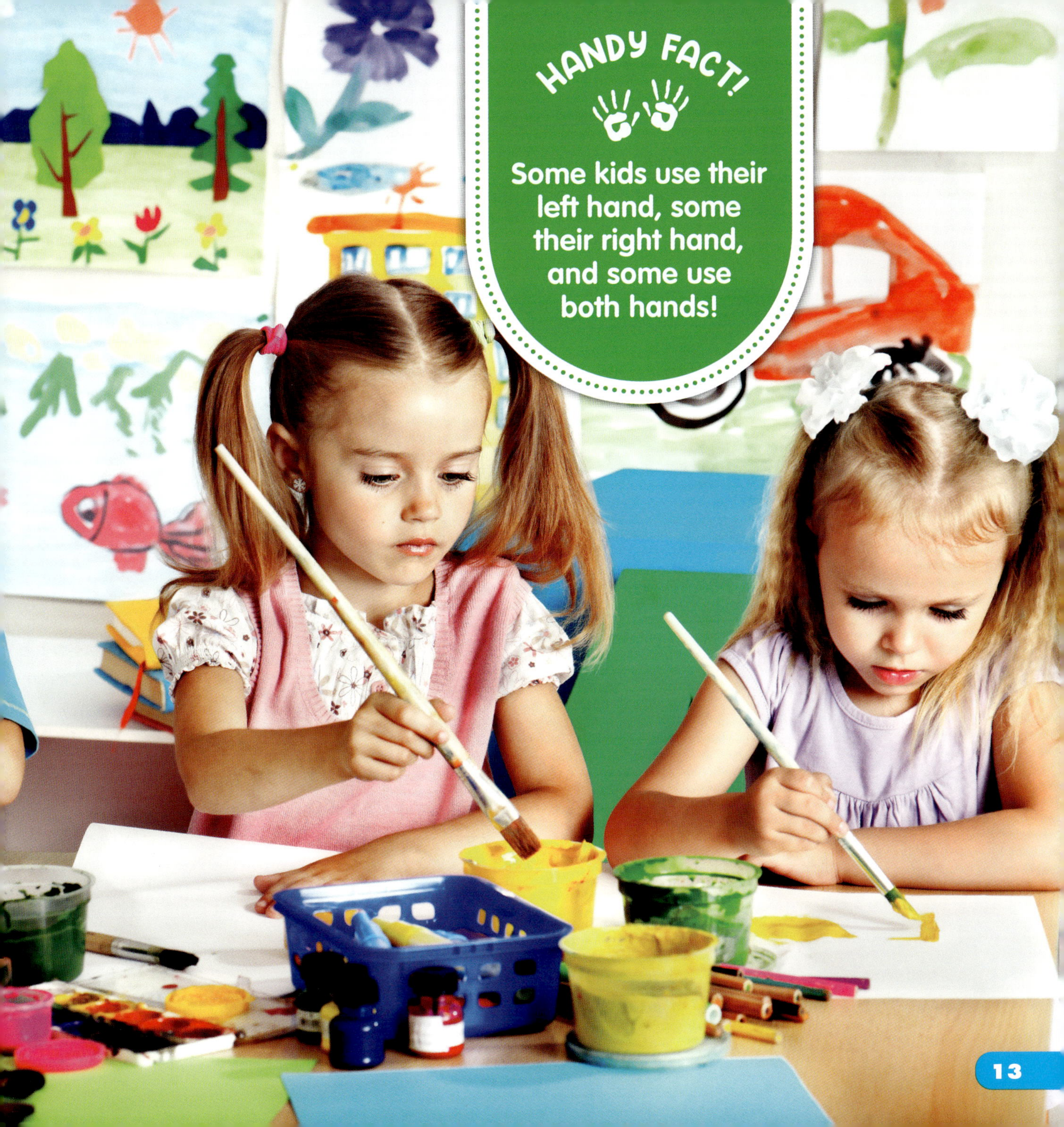

HANDY FACT!

Some kids use their left hand, some their right hand, and some use both hands!

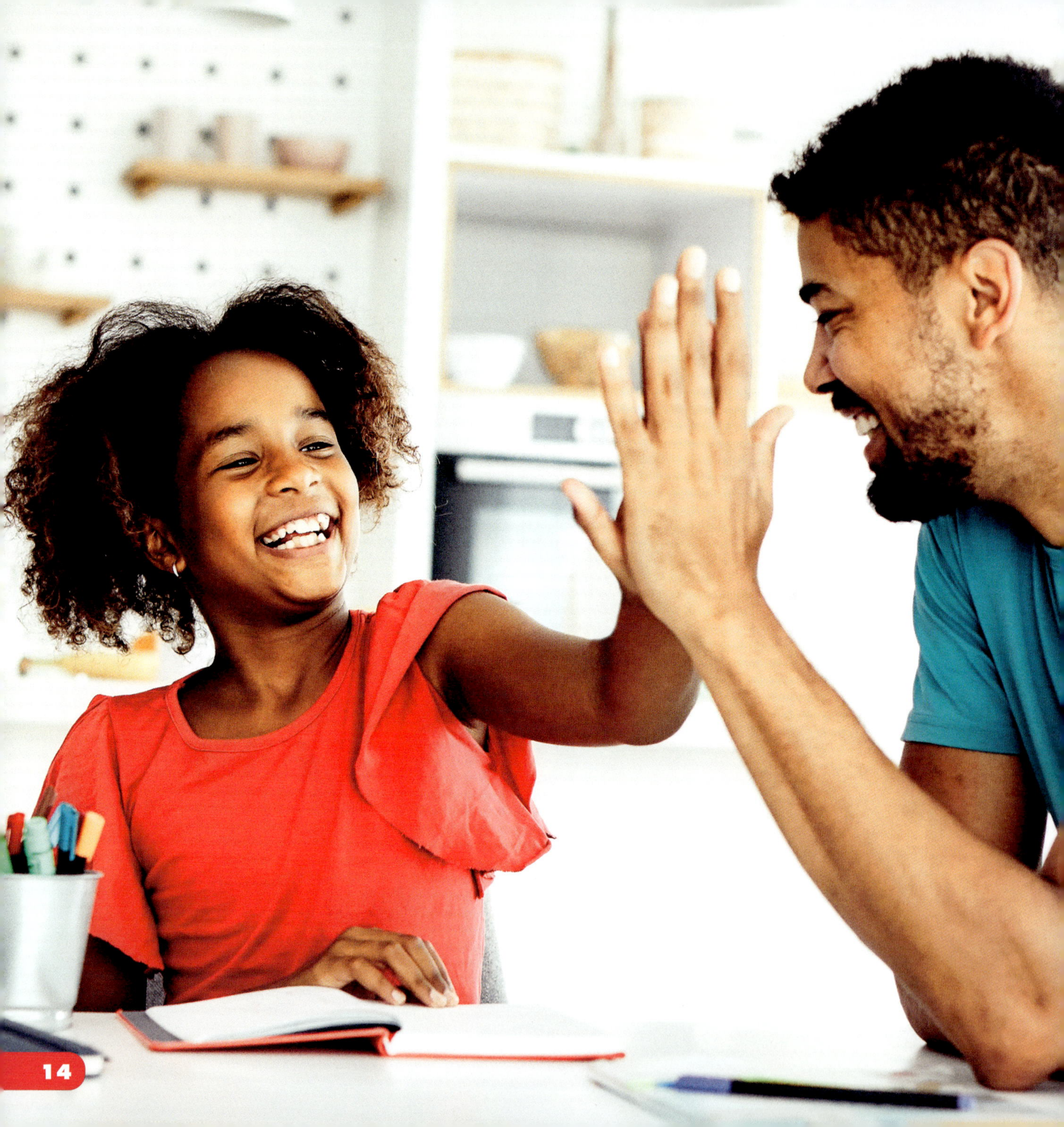

Hands wave hi.

Hands give **high fives**.

HANDY FACT!

A handshake is a way to say hello.

Work and Jobs

Hands cook food.

Hands **type** and fix.

My helping hands do big jobs.

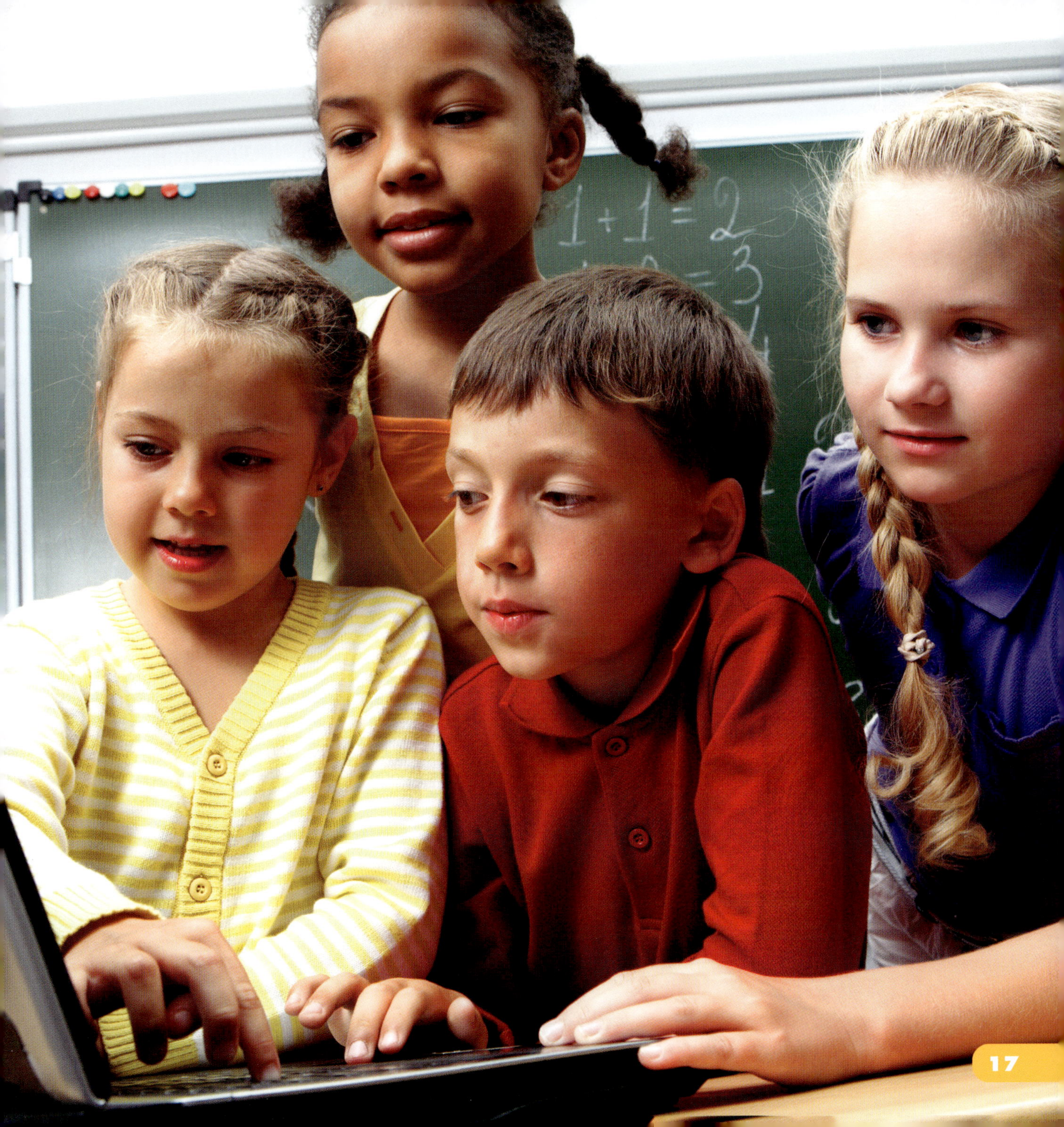
1+1=2

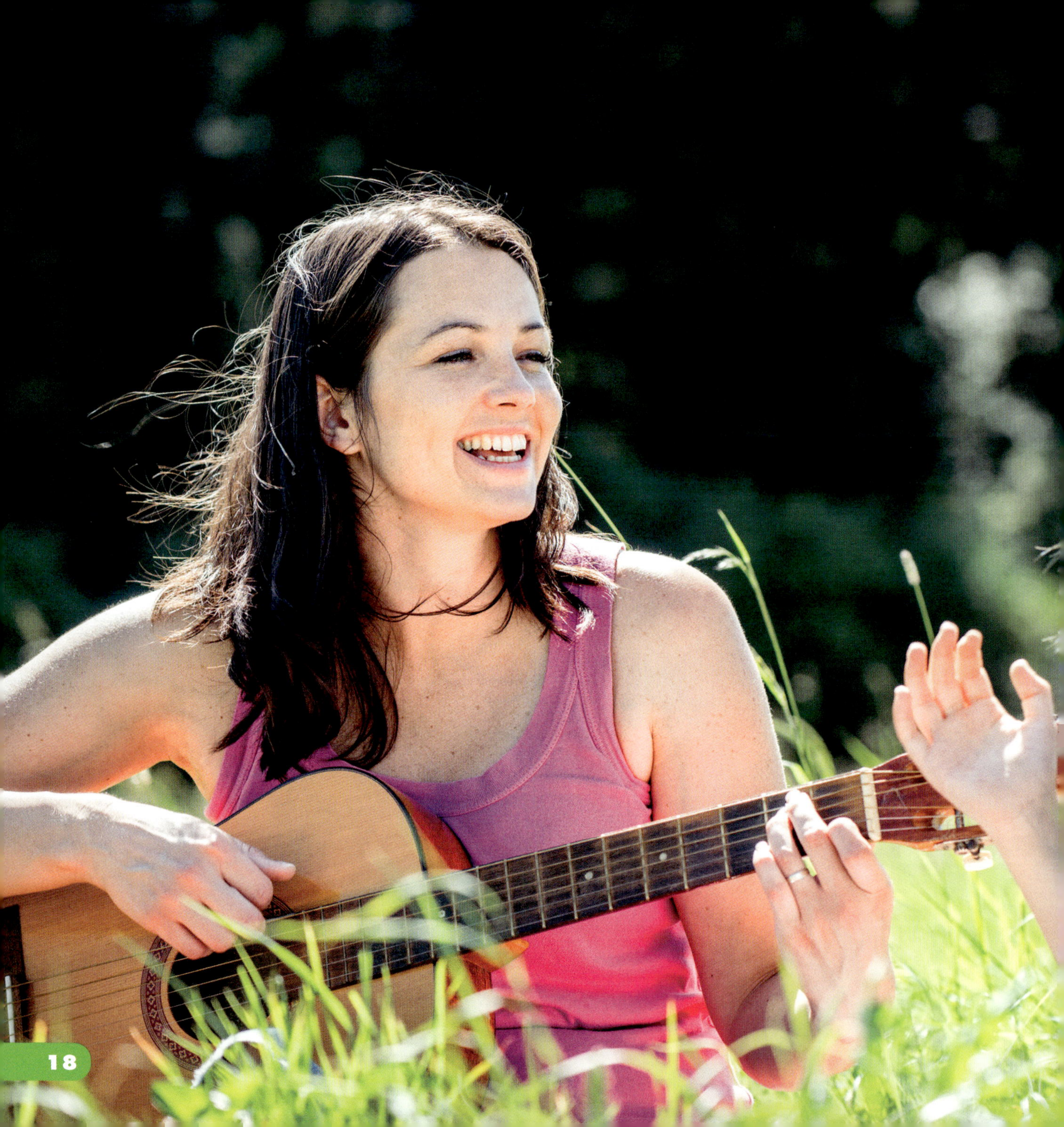

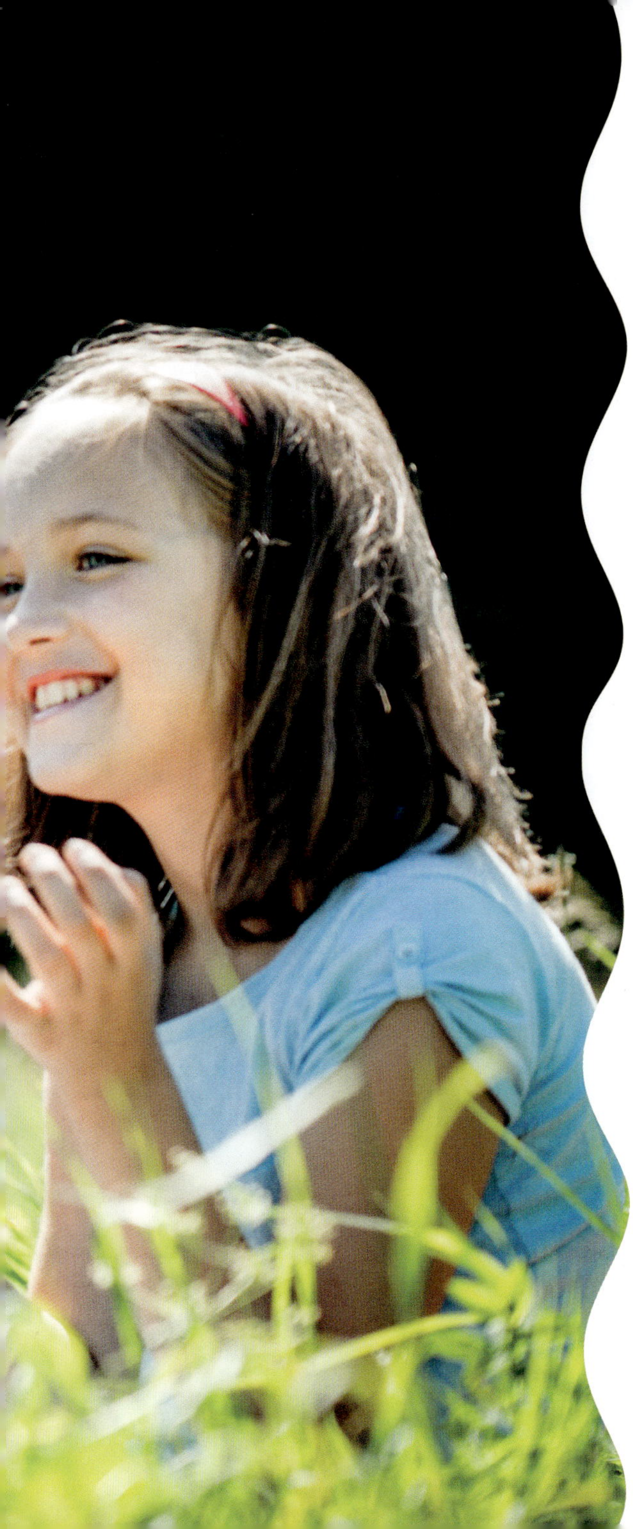

Hands clap to music.

Hands toss balls.

Resting Hands

At night, hands rest.

Tomorrow, my helping hands will help again!

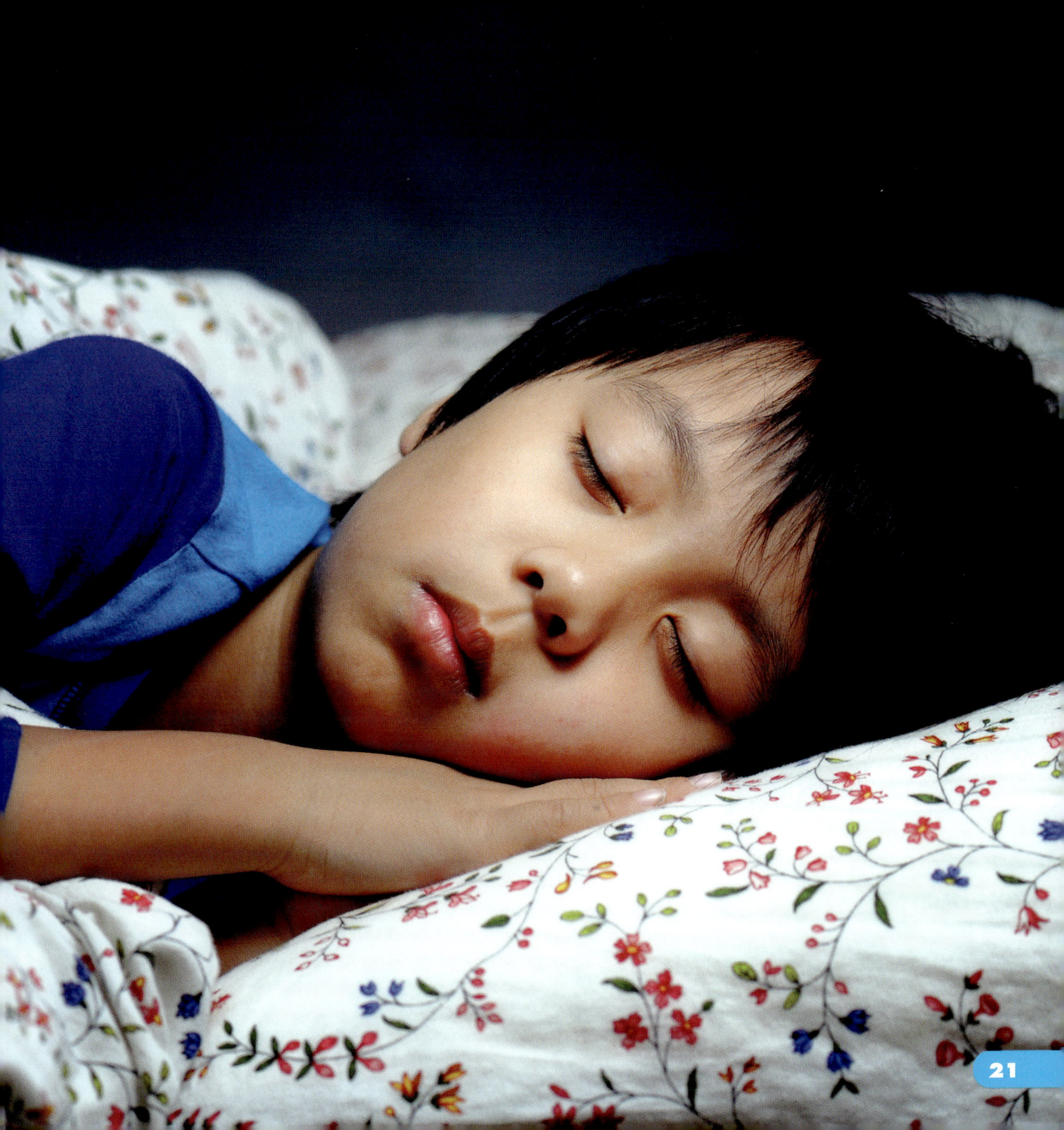

Glossary

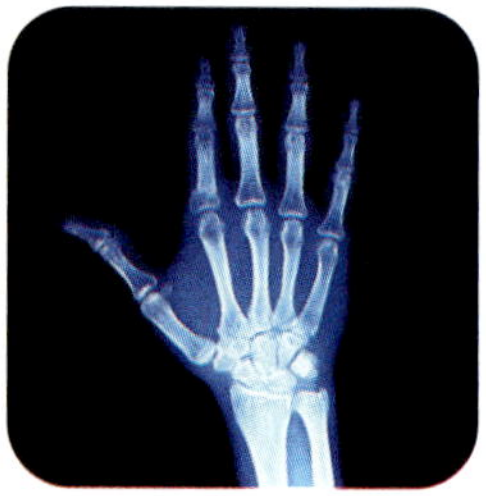

bones (bohnz) the hard parts inside your body that give it shape and support

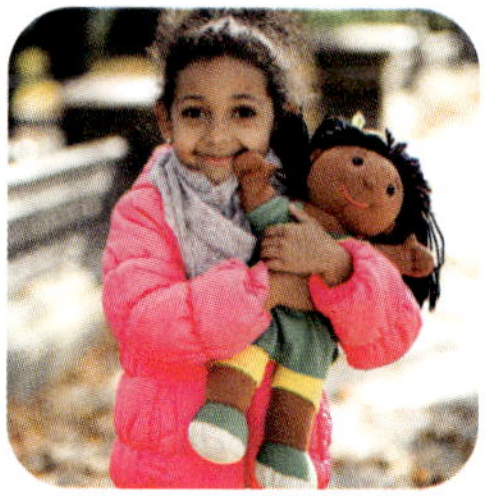

carry (KAR-ee) to take something from one place to another

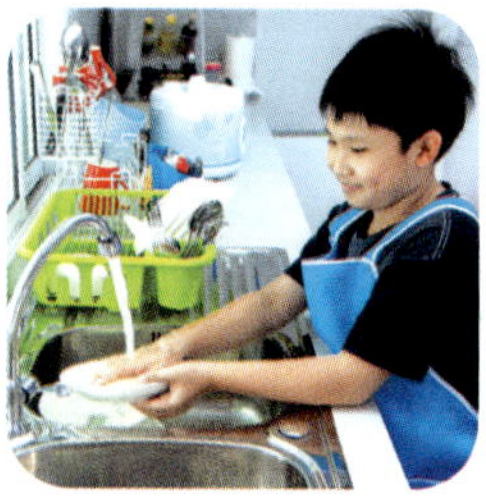

clean (kleen) to make something free of dirt

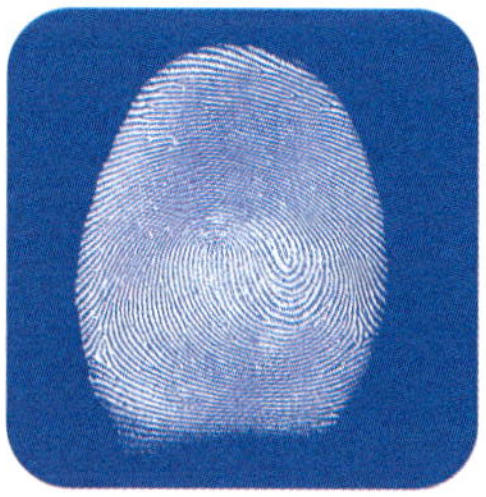

fingerprints (FING-er-prints) the tiny, unique lines on the tips of your fingers

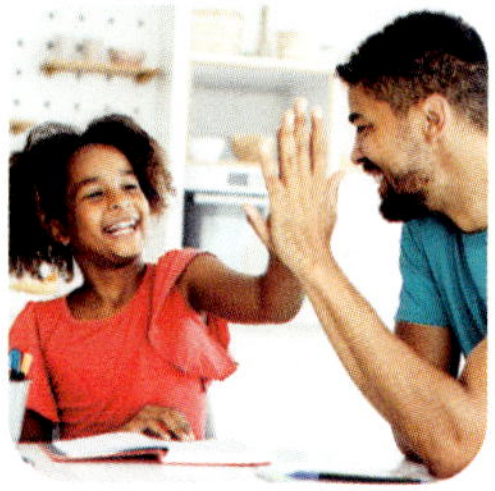

high five (hi fyv) a fun way to give someone a greeting or cheer by slapping hands

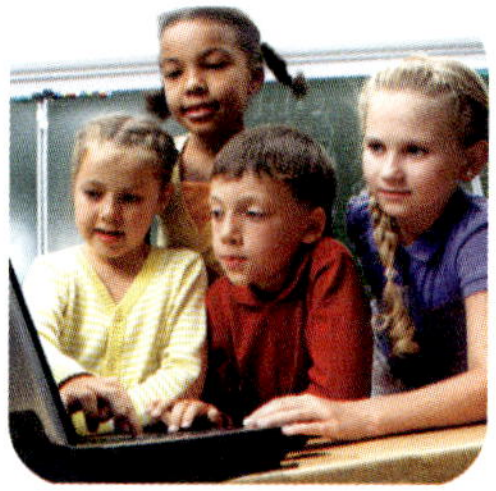

share (shair) to give some of what you have to someone else

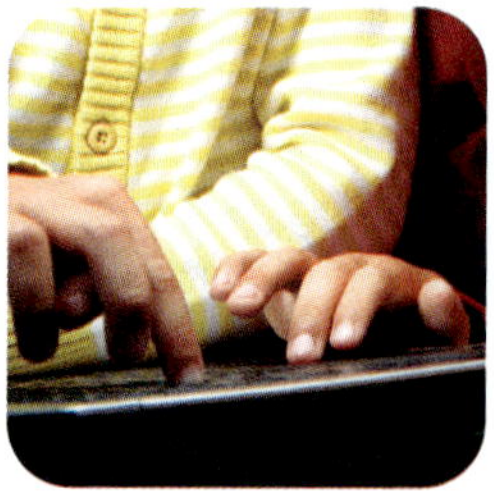

type (typ) to press letters on a keyboard to write words

Quiz: My Helping Hands

1. Do hands help you carry things?

   A. Yes B. No

2. Can helping hands wave and clap?

   A. Yes B. No

3. Do hands help you play?

   A. Yes B. No

4. Do hands need rest at night?

   A. Yes B. No

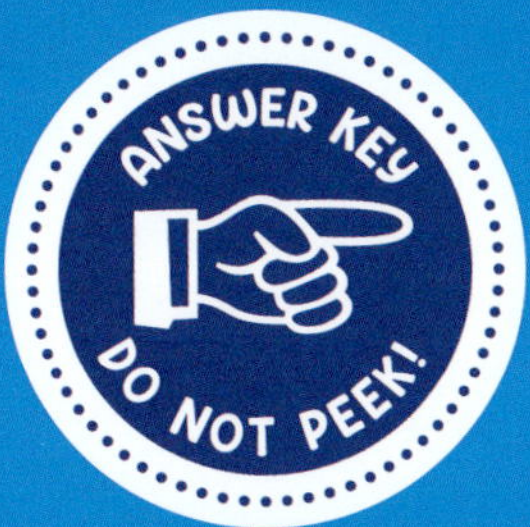

ANSWER KEY:

How many times did you answer yes?

4 Yes: Awesome! You know your hands well.

3 Yes: Great job! You learned new facts.

2 Yes: Keep reading to learn more.

1 Yes: You're just starting out. Keep going!

Further Reading

Néjib. *My Hands.* Red Comet Press, 2022.

Paquette, Ammi-Joan. *My Hands Can.* Penguin Random House, 2024.

Stutzman, Jonathan. *Soon, Your Hands.* Penguin Random House, 2023.

On the Internet

KidsSoup—Hands & Feet Activities, Rhymes, and Games
https://www.kidssoup.com/activity/hands-and-feet-activities-crafts-rhymes-and-books
This site offers creative activities like rhymes and movement games centered on hands and feet—great for gross motor development and body awareness.

The Inspired Treehouse—Going Barefoot: 10 Fun Activities for Kids
https://theinspiredtreehouse.com/going-barefoot-10-fun-activities-kids/
A playful guide packed with barefoot movement ideas—from hopping and crawling to walking on toes or heels.

Homegrown Friends—Painting with Feet
https://homegrownfriends.com/home/painting-with-feet/
A hands-on art project that invites kids to paint using their feet—engaging their sense of touch and developing gross motor skills.

Index

About the Author

Rachel Daniels is a former elementary school teacher who loves reading and discovering new things. She lives in sunny South Florida with her husband, close to her children and grandchildren. When she's not reading or writing, she enjoys playing Canasta with friends. Her goal is to make learning exciting and joyful for young readers everywhere.